*Pandemic Solutions: How to Fight COVID-19 and Other Coronaviruses*

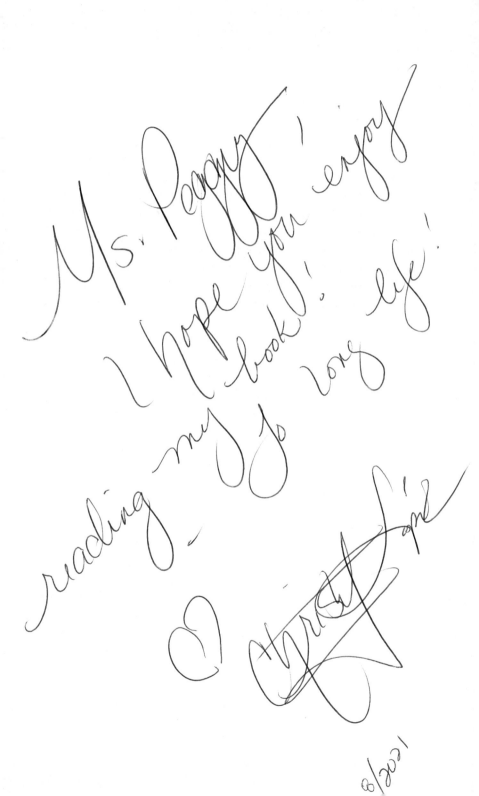

Ms. Peggy,
I hope you enjoy
reading my book! To a long life!

♡

Christyl Cope

8/30/21

# Pandemic Solutions: How to Fight COVID-19 and Other Coronaviruses

*Information, Insight, and Ingredients from Nature*

By Christy López

Ms. Christy Lopez is a highly regarded and super-talented hairstylist, makeup artist, and salon owner in the Washington, DC area. Christy has worked at every level in the beauty industry, from her first job of being a shampoo-girl to salon ownership. She has maintained a steady and racially diverse clientele throughout the years and is a master in every aspect of hairstyling. There's nothing she can't do. Clients come from near and far to have their hair styled; a few have even boarded planes or driven for hours to sit in her chair!

PurposeHouse Publishing, Columbia, Maryland.
Copyright © 2020 Christy Lopez
All rights reserved. Published 2020.

ISBN: 978-1-7329549-4-6

Published in the USA.
Cover design by PurposeHouse Publishing, all rights reserved.

# DEDICATION

When I look back over my life, my mind and heart hasten to one moment in time that assures me of God's love for me. It is the moment that cancels out every tear I've ever cried from the pain and agony of isolation, disappointment, rejection, loss, and heartbreak. It is the moment that cancels out every negative experience life has handed me—like the first step of a "solve for x" algebraic equation. It is the thought of this one moment in my life that is my will to live today, my hope for tomorrow, and why I have to believe in eternity—and that I will spend it with the gift given to me at that moment.

It is the moment that I became a mom.

This book is dedicated to my son Kyle. You are the only person this side of heaven that makes my life worth living. Thank you for always loving me and letting me know that I matter. Your encouragement feeds my soul. Your constant prayers sustain me.


You are an amazing son, and I am beyond proud of you. There has been no greater joy in my life than being your mom. I love you always.

Mom

Along the bank of the river, on this side and that, will grow all kinds of trees used for food; their leaves will not wither and their fruit will not fail. They will bear fruit every month because their water flows from the sanctuary. Their fruit will be for food, and their leaves for medicine.
(Ezekiel 47:12 KJV)
- AΩ


"All that man needs for health and healing has been provided by God in nature. The challenge of science is to find it."
- Paradesus, Philosopher, Physician, Alchemist

# CONTENTS

*Christy Lopez*

# INTRODUCTION

Never in history has any one thing captured the attention of the entire world. Yet, something invisible to the naked eye, microscopic, and measuring only four-millionths of an inch in diameter has! This something will forever be known as "The Great Equalizer!" This something is COVID-19, a Severe Acute Respiratory Syndrome-related (SARS-related) coronavirus.

The virus's name is derived from the Latin word corona, which means crown. It is aptly named due to the crown-like spikes that extend from the viral molecule. These spikes attach themselves to the lung's lining before corrupting and taking over healthy cells, leading to respiratory infection. The world has seen coronaviruses before. Meaning, other viruses have those little crown-like clusters on the end of the spikes that protrude off the viral molecule. We'll learn about a few of those as we read further. Still, none have been as swift, indiscriminate, or as deadly as this one.

COVID-19 is the official name of the infection caused by its intrusive presence. Broken down, the acronym means Corona Virus Disease-2019. Many people wonder why this condition has two names; which is it--Coronavirus or COVID-19? The answer is pretty simple. COVID-19 is the disease one develops as a result of being attacked by this particular coronavirus!

Global health organizations such as the World Health Organization (WHO), various centers for disease control, and entities track viruses, diseases, infections, and their origins. Diseases, viruses, and infections are named so that doctors, scientists, and virologists around the world will be on one accord. Imagine if the United States calls a disease "X," Canada named it "Y," while China referred to it a "Z." How confusing! That said, not every nation is on the same page for research. Scientific studies and research trials are conducted by multitudes of entities all over the world. Government scientists of nations, pharmaceutical companies, universities, and private labs are all conducting their own research. They are all employing their own technology and methodology—racing to discover breakthroughs, findings, and, eventually, a vaccine. Since COVID-19 is a virus, we are inclined to believe that there is no cure yet known to man. Much like the common cold or various iterations of influenza, which are viruses as well, they are both recurring and easily contracted as a result of exposure.

Much has been said about a second wave of viral infections after the initial crisis. History even points to its inevitability. It may come back with a vengeance because people become weary of doing what it takes to prevent becoming infected. They grow tired of the catchphrase and practice of social distancing, wearing masks, and vigorous cleaning and disinfecting. Longing for the normalcy they once enjoyed, people will begin to assemble and gather in large numbers, whether in the company of family, friends, or gathering to worship or pack out a restaurant or event venue. A resurgence could also happen because of a nexus between the cold and flu season and COVID-19.

The information presented as you read further is intended to equip you to practice holistic measures to fight this virus (and others) from a natural standpoint. It goes without saying that these measures should also be coupled with wisdom. This is not a medical journal and is in no way telling the reader to ignore established medical guidelines and protocols. Please do not forsake medical treatment when needed. And certainly, don't relax best practices in terms of hygiene and taking preventative measures. Know that this book is a guide. It is intended to inform you of what is available in nature to aid in prevention and treatment. It focuses on what's already available on the earth that was originally intended to be our medicine. This is a principal supported in holy scriptures and science! That said, this book is for everyone.

When news of an outbreak and swift spread of a deadly mystery illness emerged from Wuhan, China (in Hubei province) in late 2019, the world had no clue what was on the horizon. It quickly became clear that this was yet another coronavirus. There was an ominous warning of a cluster of these strange and extremely deadly viral infections that were presenting in the form of respiratory arrest and pneumonia. A brave Chinese doctor named Dr. Li Wenliang sounded the alarm. In a closed group within WeChat, an online chatroom, he told his medical school colleagues about this peculiar epidemic resembling SARS (severe acute respiratory syndrome) that was causing patients to be quarantined.

Most of us, as a normal course of a conversation about current events or as a responsible citizen raising questions about local goings-on, would have done the same. However, the most likely reason for the good doctor to have spoken up about what he saw happening is that he was upholding the Hippocratic oath. Unfortunately, the Chinese government didn't see things that way. Dr. Li was found, summoned by police (along with seven others), and interrogated. With the full weight of (non-democratic) government officials in China bearing down on him, he was coerced into signing a statement admitting that he was guilty of spreading lies and rumors about the looming viral crisis. The entire world now knows that he was, in fact, telling the truth! Sadly, on February 7, 2020, Dr. Li Wenliang died from the very coronavirus he warned the world about. At that time, it was called SARS CoV-2. He left behind a pregnant wife and a young son. He was thirty-three years old.

As the now named COVID-19 virus spread throughout the world, scientists and physicians were making solid discoveries regarding its nature, symptoms, and effects. No sooner than these discoveries were adopted by the medical community and citizens globally, the findings and truths about the virus began to change. It was initially believed that the virus did not affect children. But it soon began to infect and claim the lives of children and infants. By late April 2020, children and young adults began to present with a strange inflammatory Kawasaki-like illness. Parents noticed bluish lips, a red rash covering their children's bodies that were running extremely high fevers. Some children experienced respiratory distress and cardiac arrest. Healthy adults with no underlying health conditions or co-morbidities (such as diabetes, hypertension, or heart disease, to name a few) were thought to be all but exempt from the effects of COVID-19. But it is not so. Healthy doctors and nurses contracted COVID-19. Many died. On May 14, 2020, virologist, epidemiologist, and NBC news medical correspondent, Dr. Joseph Fair, announced that he had also fallen victim to the very virus that he had given counsel about. A far cry from the notion that the virus (now pandemic) would only adversely affect the sick and the elderly. We realized that even those who had not travelled to and from Wuhan, China, were at risk. As previously stated, COVID-19 would become "The Great Equalizer."

It is imperative that every citizen around the globe remain vigilant in their fight against contracting COVID-19. Many places hard hit with extremely high death tolls such as Italy, Spain, and the United States have begun to see high mortality rates taper off, though there were still hotspots as of July 2020. Native American communities in North America are especially hard hit. The rate of infection and death among Native Americans is extremely high based on their actual population, so their per capita percentage makes their communities a hotspot. As of June, and well into July 2020, Brazil in South America is leading the world in deaths and infections as their defiant president continues to pretend that there is no real pandemic at hand. From the beginning of this crisis, he has argued the contrary to what medical science and the obvious mass loss of life have proven. This pandemic is real! On June 6, 2020, the Brazilian government made a stunning move that goes beyond any reasonable comprehension. They decided to stop publishing the numbers of infections and deaths, and they removed all history of daily reports of infections and deaths from government websites. This is not just a national travesty for Brazil, but also a brazen injustice to the world. History will now never know or reflect the full scope of this pandemic on a global scale with hidden and unreported information. What gross incompetence!

It is critical to be vigilant and do all that needs to be done to take care of oneself and their families. It is essential that each person do all they can to stop the spread of this deadly virus to others, and this book aims to help you do so.

The information presented in this book is designed to aid in the process of self-care from a holistic perspective. Herbs and spices and the manner of preparation of some foods have been a hallmark to health and healing from the beginning of time. Across the globe, humanity used what nature provided for healing and treatment long before modern medicine and pharmaceutical companies ever existed. Ages, even centuries before chemical compound remedies (drugs) were designed, tested, and pushed onto the sick as treatments for ailments and diseases, nature already had the cure.

Cure is a word that is hardly ever used in modern medicine. Cures run counter to capitalism! If people are cured from what ails them, doctors and big pharma aren't able to profit (benefit financially) from those people. Therefore, we now live in a culture where diseases and health issues are being managed. Diseases are not being cured! People are not being healed! There is even the conditioning of the mind that robs people of the hope for healing because they are told that there is no cure.

I have designed this book, *Pandemic Solutions: How to Fight COVID-19 and Other Coronaviruses*, as a tool to share some of the remedies found in nature that are readily available to help your body prevent and fight off viruses, bacteria, fungus, and inflammation. It explores natural herbs and spices to add to one's diet, as well as a few foods one can consume to assist in enabling the body to fight to remain healthy. Again, let me reiterate that this is information, not a medical journal or in any way suggests that its reader avoid seeking medical treatment.

Stay wise. Stay healthy!

# CHAPTER 1: WHAT IS A VIRUS?

A virus is a submicroscopic agent that brings about the infection of a living thing by corrupting and replicating itself inside of (and taking over) healthy cells. It is made up of genetic material, Deoxyribonucleic acid (DNA) or Ribonucleic acid (RNA), and contains its own genetic instructions (sequencing) to duplicate itself.

In and of itself, a virus is inert. It is not even alive but gets its power from its host, which is alive. Humans, animals, and plants can all become a host and are susceptible to viral infections. Needless to say, no host of a virus, whether it be deadly or survivable, is a willing host. I dare to say that no thing, and certainly, no one wants to be invaded.

Isn't it amazing to know that something that isn't even alive can wreak so much havoc on the living?

As we learn how to navigate the world with the coronavirus, which leads to COVID-19, it is essential to learn about virology, the study of viruses. Obviously, such a small guidebook will in no way be sufficient for the comprehension necessary to make one an expert. Medical students who study virology usually marry their studies with a focus on epidemiology. And they spend many years in college to earn a doctorate degree. Some do so to become a specialist in this field as a Medical Doctor (MD). Others continue in this area of study to earn a PhD (Doctor of Philosophy) and focus on medical research and development. Either way, they are driven by a passion and educational dedication that takes years. That's much more time than these writings could ever delve into in any substantive way.

That said, it is still important to have a basic understanding of what a virus is and how it works.

There has been much speculation about the origins of the coronavirus. The conclusion has been that COVID-19 came through animal to human transmission. Many theorize that bats handled or consumed from a wet market, offering live animals for sale, in Wuhan, China are the initial outbreak source. We won't go down that "rabbit hole" because there are so many theories out there. However, it is important to note that animal-to-human (not human-to-animal) arguments have been bandied about within the research community. And there have been reports of a few cases of household pets—dogs and cats—as well as a few big cats such as lions and tigers in the Bronx Zoo that have tested positive for COVID-19. It is safe to say that more research needs to be done in that arena.

Still, understanding human susceptibility to viruses isn't a new quest. There are many known viruses that science fully understands. The common cold and flu are examples. The flu, short for influenza, is a virus that attacks the respiratory system. It is spread through droplets from coughs, sneezes, airborne saliva, and contact with contaminated surfaces that make their way into one's mucus membranes, the eyes, nose, or mouth.

Influenza has several iterations. Quite a few strains of influenza exist. The most common are Influenza A and B. There are also C and D strains. A few strains have also hit the United States over the last ten to fifteen years, such as Avian Influenza (bird flu) and Swine Influenza (swine flu). As their names imply, they are flu strains that originated from wild birds and poultry, and pigs, respectively. Remember, some viruses are known to be transferrable from animals to humans.

Highly contagious, the Norovirus is introduced through contaminated food or water. Equally contagious and extremely crippling is the Rotavirus. This virus is contracted from fecal-oral contact such as ingesting food or drink tainted with or handled by hands that are unclean or other contacts with hands with traces of feces that somehow enter one's mouth. Both viruses cause similar symptoms such as fever, nausea, vomiting, abdominal pain, and diarrhea, which may lead to dehydration.

There are many other kinds of viruses, including Herpes Simplex Viruses 1 and 2 and HIV, the virus that causes Acquired Immune Deficiency Syndrome (AIDS), that are transmitted by sexual or skin-to-skin contact. These are well understood due to years of research and medical treatment development, including anti-viral and anti-retroviral medications.

During the COVID-19 era and the ensuing quick spread and high mortality numbers, much has been said about the influenza pandemic that swept the globe over 100 years ago. It is believed to have started in France but was given the moniker the Spanish flu because Spain's news media was the first to report its onset and spread. This pandemic lasted for a little over two years and claimed the lives of an estimated 20,000,000 to 50,000,000 worldwide. Yes, you read that correctly—twenty to fifty million! Some believe that the death toll may have claimed as many as 100,000,000 lives. That was about 3% of the world's population at that time.

Several factors contributed to the mass loss of life. Contemplate the following: This pandemic was happening during World War I. The patent for aspirin, trademarked by Bayer in 1899, expired in 1917, and other companies tried to duplicate the medication in haste. The US Surgeon General at that time, Rupert Blue, the US Navy, and the Journal of the American Medical Association all recommended the use of aspirin to treat the flu. Medical professionals advised taking up to thirty grams per day. It was a dose now known to be toxic! Citizens began to show signs and symptoms of aspirin poisoning. Deaths increased rapidly. More US Servicemen died from the Spanish flu than from the war!

It is important to note that the comparison of COVID-19 to the Spanish flu isn't hyperbole. The parallels are shocking, considering developments, modernization, and medical research and advancements over the past century. Over 100 years have passed, yet the extreme steps that have had to be taken to deal with coronavirus in 2020 are identical. Using New York as the example, just as was the case during the Spanish flu in 1918, the state was completely shut down in 2020, except for essential businesses such as grocery stores, pharmacies, and hospitals. On March 20, 2020, New York Governor Andrew Cuomo issued a state-wide stay-at-home order for all residents of the state apart from essential workers. Only first responders, doctors, nurses and hospital staff, grocery, and pharmacy workers, and what soon became overworked funeral workers were exempted from the order.

Restaurants were permitted to open but were limited to only a few workers and were only allowed to deliver or have patrons pick up food. The subway and metro systems were limited to ridership of only essential workers but were eventually closed completely at night for the arduous task of disinfecting trains and buses. All retail shopping was closed. The stay-at-home order was issued so that people would not be out and about spreading and contracting the virus, just as in 1918. Those who had to travel to and from work or necessary shopping were admonished to stay no less than six feet away from others, much like they were in 1918. Sadly but necessarily, no visitors were allowed into hospitals or nursing homes. Those who perished died alone. Some families were only able to watch loved ones slip away if nurses were with the patient and compassionate enough to reach out to the family on cell phones or tablets. Bodies of the dead, nearly 1000 per day at the peak of the pandemic, were piled high in refrigerated trailer trucks. If families failed to claim their loved ones remains within fourteen days, bodies were sent to Potters Field on Hart Island in New York to be buried unceremoniously in a mass grave. Morgue workers and the National Guard worked tirelessly, digging and covering grave trenches. The indignities of this tragedy were unfathomable yet were suffered none the less.

Because of the gross number of deceased, coupled with the gravity of the virus, funerals became nothing more than drive-by graveside services or memorials with no more than ten persons allowed to attend. Because funeral homes were overwhelmed, Gov. Cuomo made a public appeal for licensed funeral directors from other states to come to New York to help with the insurmountable number of bodies. These unprecedented times called for such desperate measures.

This is what a virus is. This is what a virus can do.

New York was shut down for just over three months.

# CHAPTER 2: IN THE BEGINNING

M any early writings and sacred texts of various faiths and belief systems point to the use of spices, herbs, and their leaves for healing purposes. Many will be surprised to learn that most of the herbs and spices available today are the same ones used over 2000 years ago for food and medicine.

When it comes to adding a holistic approach to helping one's body prevent and fight off viral infections, the age-old phrase "what's old is new again" rings true. COVID-19 has presented many reasons and the urgency for people to identify ways to guard themselves against its effects. Medical interventions are literally the "practice" of medicine, as there is still no agreed-upon course of treatment for COVID-19 in the medical community. Neither are there any pharmaceutical therapies that are promising in any way. The singular truth that everyone in the medical community does agree on is that the development of a vaccine is critical!

Until then and even after a successful vaccine has been developed, building and maintaining one's health and immune system will be predicated upon holistic, homeopathic, and natural sources. The signs are already frighteningly clear as the supply of even what's being tried on patients as medical (drug) treatments have been running out quite regularly during this pandemic. They are running out and not being able to be fulfilled or produced in a manner where the supply meets the demand.

Just contemplate for a minute if you or your loved one is a patient, having fallen victim to COVID-19 or any other crippling virus. Now imagine being told that any interventions, whether proven or trial, are all gone. There is no more. It is back-ordered or yet to even be produced. As a worst-case scenario, imagine learning that there is a matter of red tape involved. For example, politics or bureaucratic wrangling of some kind would eclipse desperately needed medical care. These are sobering thoughts, indeed.

The days of blissful ignorance and blind trust in our country's systems to do what is right for its citizens are long gone. Our healthcare system has been ailing for a long, long time, and is now on a ventilator itself. Power-drunk and clumsy government officials are poised to trip over the cord. People must take it upon themselves to be intentional about ways to become and remain optimally healthy. This has never been more abundantly clear. There is hope for all of us to be able to do just that. The hope is found in nature.

As stated before, since the beginning of time, much has been written about what is available from the earth to be used for health and healing. Going forward, you will see that pretty much all faith traditions have this in common. Let's learn of a few.

The Holy Bible, the sacred text of the Christian faith, speaks much about healing. In the passage of Mark 10:46-52, a man named Bartimaeus, who had become blind, was healed by Jesus. In John 9:1-12, there is an unnamed man who was blind from birth. Here, the passage tells of how Jesus used two of the most unlikely elements to make a salve for his eyes that indeed gave him sight.

There was a woman who suffered from her medical condition for twelve years. Known in the Bible as "the woman with the issue of blood," she knew and understood that the power of Jesus was the only thing that could truly heal her. On the day he passed through her city, the woman—weak yet resilient, desperate but determined, and now poor from having spent all of her money on doctors—decided to fight her way through the dense crowd that surrounded him. She managed to crawl and get only close enough to grab just the edge of his garment. This bold move changed her life!

Jesus knew that although there were scores of people touching him as he walked through the multitude, that only one of the many drew healing virtue from him. Jesus stopped and asked a question—a rhetorical one, as he already knew the answer. "Who touched me?" People thought that was an odd ask, considering how many people were touching him. He then goes on to explain that although many people were touching him, there was one that he knew had been healed. Nervous and vulnerable, the woman spoke up. Jesus's response to her was epic! He told her to "go in peace and to be of good cheer—your faith has made you whole." She was healed immediately! The account of this miracle can be found in three different places in the Bible, Matthew 9:20-22, Mark 5: 25-34, and Luke 8:43-48. In some translations of the Bible, the scripture reads, "your faith

Although most references in the Bible are about healing through miracles performed by Jesus Christ, some scriptures specifically speak to natural remedies. Ezekiel 47:12 NIV tells us:

> *Fruit trees of all kinds will grow on both banks of the river. Their leaves will not wither, nor will their fruit fail. Every month they will bear fruit, because the water from the sanctuary flows to them. Their fruit will serve for food, and their leaves for healing. Some translations read, "and their leaves for medicine.*

The same is mentioned again in Revelation 22:2. In Isaiah 38:21, Isaiah gave Hezekiah's servants instructions, saying, "Make an ointment of figs and spread it over the boil, and Hezekiah will recover." This account may also be found in 2 Kings 20:1-7.

Cinnamon, frankincense, myrrh, saffron, nard, cumin, and coriander, in addition to the leaves and stems of various annual and perennial plants, were used in a medicinal capacity in biblical accounts. Garlic and its leaves and blossoms were used, as was wine and honey.

In other cultures and faith traditions, natural remedies were not only used but also were celebrated. There were even songs sung about them. One of the world's oldest healing systems practices the balance of mind, body, and spirit. It hinges on the premise of maintaining good health, not fighting disease. It is called Ayurvedic medicine. Hindu writings have well documented Ayurvedic prophylactics and treatments. Much may be learned about these practices by reading the sacred texts of Hindu culture, The Four Vedas.

The Rig Veda, in particular, chronicles an abundance of Ayurvedic solutions for just about every area of life. Songs and hymns pay homage to many herbs believed to hold within them the cures to all diseases. In the Rig Veda, the hymn called The Healing Plants is the most popular of all songs. Books of Sushrut and Charaka tout hundreds of herbs. Charaka, (born in 300 BC in the Punjab region if India) is regarded as the "Indian Father of Medicine." Ayurvedic medicine and therapies have become extremely popular throughout the western world. They are extremely popular in body wellness services in fine spas in the United States.

Some readily available spices one can incorporate on their journey to health and boost the body's ability to fight viruses are turmeric, cardamom, licorice root, coriander, ginger, and cumin. Bitter melon, gooseberries, aloe, and holy basil are excellent things to add to one's diet as well. There are literally hundreds of herbs, spices, and food remedies that should be explored; these popular ones barely scratch the surface.

In Judaism, The Talmud speaks of various natural sources for health solutions. Plants, fruits, vegetables, and spices are touted for their ability to treat various ailments. Some are even regarded as cures. The Talmud even touches on some natural solutions for increasing virility and inducing temporary sterility, preventing conception! Yes--boosting male fertility, performance, stamina, and even birth control was written about as early as the Fourth Century. In addition to the treatment that stops hemorrhaging in the body, other specific health concerns are addressed as well. Eye conditions, intestinal worms, bowel issues, liver conditions, skin diseases, scurvy, blood pressure, and other blood conditions, to name a handful, are addressed. Pomegranates, olives, dates, garlic, beets, hyssop, spinach beet, and plants and spices such as saffron and cinnamon were used as medicine and for food. Frankincense and myrrh were widely used as both have healing properties. But frankincense is also known as a sedative. It is incredibly necessary for extremely painful sicknesses. Wine was also used for those extremely pained in sickness.

It is important to note that the holy books of Judaism are the Torah and the Tanakh; the first five books of the Bible, and subsequently, most of the books of the Old Testament, respectively. The Talmud, however, is an extremely revered book of extensive rabbinical theological studies and conclusions (summaries) of the same.

Tibetan Buddhist medicine is central to the preservation of this far Eastern culture. Tibetan herbalists have been using specially curated herb teas for generations for health and the balance of life. The book of the Four Medical Tantras is where one can learn about these practices.

The COVID-19 pandemic has caused people around the entire world to think about and reevaluate healthcare, and the need to be intentionally proactive about their own health. Certainly, natural methods are being considered.

Learning about ancient, holistic methodologies and those based on faith traditions that have stood the test of time may prove beneficial these days. Although the aforementioned information isn't a full exegesis, it does provide the framework from which one can dig deeper to learn of the natural health practices of cultures and faith communities. It may prove to be, at the very least, helpful, and at best critical in helping people fight against

COVID-19 and other viruses.

*Christy Lopez*

# CHAPTER 3: FOOD FOR THOUGHT

L et's admit it. One of life's most simple pleasures is food! It is also one of the guilty pleasures of over-indulgence for those that—well, over-indulge. Whether one is poor and destitute in a famine-stricken village or uber-wealthy, living in extreme opulence with untold fortunes, everyone looks forward to mealtime. One could presume that hungry children barely able to muster enough strength to wave away the flies that surround them (that we see on charity organizations TV commercials) must live for the moment they get a nutritious meal and a cool refreshing drink. Likewise, the rich and powerful make sport of dining at the most luxurious and expensive restaurants in the world; they consume meals consisting of many courses prepared by renowned chefs. Business deals, mergers, and acquisitions often begin in fine steak houses or private dining rooms in members' only establishments. Food and drink are part and parcel to "sealing the deal."

From the old days of the ringing of the triangle dinner bell at chuckwagons to mom's dinner call, summoning children from the cul-de-sac, backyards, and playing fields across the globe, food is and has always been central to life!

We live in an age where food choice and food waste among the haves is as prevalent as food insecurity for the have nots. What's largely ignored these days is the wisdom in making healthy choices concerning what to eat. The focus is no longer on eating to live or to nourish and heal our bodies. This is evident in the rates of obesity (even morbid obesity), diabetes, and many other chronic health issues brought on by poor food choice and consumption of gross amounts of sugar, salt, preservatives, and processed foods. What is also evident (medically verified) is that most health issues can be remedied—even eliminated—by healthy eating and adjusting one's diet to create the balance needed for what ails an individual's body. Those who struggle with health concerns and obesity should consult a physician or healthcare provider. Some health issues are complex and may not get better by healthy food choices and intentional eating alone.

For years, the food pyramid in all its iterations has provided a guide for how to eat for optimal health. It takes the approach of indicating how many servings of meat, dairy, whole grains, and fruits and vegetables one needs to be healthy. It is safe to say that surely the guide is just that—a guide.

It is a recommendation from one school of thought. Consider that many people in the world don't even eat meat or any animal products. Some people don't consume dairy. Knowing this, it is safe to say that there needs to be more conversations and information presented about what and how to eat to be healthy than just a predominant American perspective being taught from the food pyramid theory.

Much thought should be given to the ways we can adjust our diets and how we should eat and drink for our health. Making necessary changes now to improve our eating habits by consuming healthy and meaningful foods and drinks will play a key role in our bodies being able to fight off sickness. This really is the time to be intentional about consuming healthy, organic (non-GMO) foods that have immune-boosting properties and are high in vitamins, minerals, and proteins. Consider taking some non-GMO supplements or adding healthy smoothies to your diet. When done right, smoothies can be excellent meal replacements. Find ways to add purposeful herbs and spices to your smoothies, drinks, and meals. Eliminate junk foods, soft drinks, sugars, salt, and processed foods from your diet.

Healthy eating is critical now more than ever, as we need to do all we can to fortify our bodies to fight off COVID-19, other coronaviruses, and diseases.

# CHAPTER 4: FERMENTED FOODS

T here are many natural things on the earth we can employ to build up our immune systems. As we know, herbs and spices play a huge role. However, there is one particularly important food category that is not talked about much. Yet these foods provide many benefits to the body that should no longer be ignored. It is time to become educated about and begin to consume fermented foods!

So, what are fermented foods? What exactly are their benefits? Well, first things first. Let's define fermentation.

Fermentation (of food) is the process by which carbohydrates are converted to alcohol or organic acids using yeast or bacteria (microorganisms) under anaerobic conditions (lack of oxygen) for the desired effect.

One might wonder how adding fermented foods to their diet may help in preventing or fighting COVID-19 or other coronaviruses. That's a fair enough question to raise, considering that we have been conditioned to believe that pharmaceutical drugs—pills and other medicines—are the answer to all that ails us. This conditioning is exactly the desired outcome; it is precisely the "return on the investment" on obscene amounts of money pharmaceutical companies spend.

Ponder this: Between 1998 and 2005, pharmaceutical companies spent 900 million dollars on lobbying. Contrast that number with the 300 million dollars they spent on lobbying in 2019 alone. One-third of the amount of money that had previously taken seven years to spend was doled out in one year!

Pharmaceutical companies made payouts to doctors to the tune of 20 billion dollars. They spent six billion dollars in drug ads in 2018. It's safe to say that throwing millions of dollars at politicians, billions at doctors, and more billions to run constant ads in all forms of media is most certainly designed to condition people to trust the narrative and the drugs being pushed. In contrast to the ever-increasing amount of sickness and diseases that people are suffering from, these staggering figures are enough to cause one to believe that something isn't quite right. Practicing doctors getting compensated from pharmaceutical companies whose drugs they then push is completely unethical! As stated before, cures run counter to capitalism!

A healthy immune system is critical to one's overall health. Fermented foods provide several significant benefits that need to be touted as we look to do all we can to fortify our bodies during this pandemic and beyond. Some of the benefits of fermented foods are:

• They improve digestive health.

• They fight off bad bacteria in your gut with good bacteria. Good gut health helps the body fight off infections such as the common cold.

• These foods restore gut health and balance after taking antibiotics.

• Rich in probiotics, fermented foods help to alleviate symptoms of a common digestive disorder called Irritable Bowel Syndrome (IBS), as well as bloating, gas, and diarrhea.

• They help the body produce certain vitamins needed for good health, including Vitamins B, K, and C, to be exact.

In addition, fermented foods provide the body with iron and zinc and aids in decreasing belly fat and contributing to weight loss. There is also evidence of reducing blood pressure and lowering cholesterol, especially Low-density Lipoproteins (LDL), the bad cholesterol.

There are also some fermented drinks to consider adding to your diet.

It's common knowledge that alcoholic beverages, especially beer and wines, result from fermentation. Grains such as barley, hops, and wheat, and various kinds of grapes (or other fruits) are mixed with varying amounts of other ingredients and fermented under varying temperatures and amounts of time to produce beer and wine, respectively. The material of the container it ferments in, and the variables of ingredients, time, and temperature are critical in producing the desired product. Many a debate has been had about whether alcohol can be good for the body versus the many ways we know it can be detrimental to the body. This is a decision that adults must weigh for themselves. There is no significant data on the effects consumption of alcohol may have on contracting coronaviruses or how it may affect people with or those who have resolved from COVID-19. However, there is plenty of information on how red wines can be beneficial when consumed in moderation. In no way is this a suggestion to drink alcohol as a treatment or remedy. For those who choose to drink, red wine is probably a safer bet because of its other known benefits. For those who consume alcohol, please drink responsibly; do not drink and drive.

Since there isn't a huge focus on the benefits of fermented foods and drinks at large, this pandemic presents a great time for individuals to familiarize themselves with and to consider adding some to their diet. Keep in mind that some items are culturally prevalent and may be found in the ethnic foods' aisles in grocery stores. The popularity of Kombucha, a cold tea drink, makes it easy to find. And it is usually featured prominently in the refrigerated drinks section of most stores.

The unprecedented era of COVID-19 has presented a unique challenge for us all to be vigilant and creative in our approach to managing our personal health. For those that choose to incorporate fermented foods and drinks, the following is a list of the most popular ones.

- Sauerkraut
- Tempeh
- Natto
- Miso
- Kimchi

- Yogurt
- Olives
- Salami
- Sourdough bread
- Some Cheeses
- Kefir
- Kombucha
- Beer
- Wine

The singular most popular fermented product that offers myriad health benefits is none other than apple cider vinegar. Commonly referred to as ACV, organic apple cider vinegar with the "mother," the cloudy looking strands in the bottle, is best. The "mother" is a network of good bacteria, enzymes, amino acids, and probiotics that bond together. It is healthy and safe to consume. Pasteurized ACV has had the mother removed and is therefore thought of as not as good, but is certainly more aesthetically pleasing, as it is not cloudy.

History supports that as far back as 400 BC in Greece, Hippocrates, the father of medicine, treated his patients with ACV. He used it to treat sores, wounds of all kinds, and to fight colds and infections. Even then, it was known to be anti-microbial and anti-fungal and to have healing properties.

Today, there are many common uses for ACV that yield positive medical results. It has been proven that ACV reduces blood sugar levels, aids significantly in weight loss, and improves digestion issues, as it is a probiotic. It is known to slow down the reproduction of cancer cells. Heart disease risks are lowered, as

ACV lowers blood pressure (hypertension) and cholesterol (overall, triglycerides, and LDL). Apple cider vinegar provides many more health and wellness benefits that one should research, along with the other fermented foods listed.

Care should be exercised when consuming ACV, as the acidity isn't good for the enamel of teeth. As with any serious medical concerns, use wisdom, and seek advice from your health care provider.

# Chapter 5: GMOs vs. Organic: Genetically Modified Organisms vs. Real Food

I f it looks like a duck, swims like a duck, and quacks like a duck, then it's probably a duck. Right? Well, not so!

In 1738, a Frenchman named Jacques de le Vaucanson created a mechanical duck that was able to flap its wings, eat, drink, digest food, and quack like a real live duck. This mechanical duck was even able to excrete digested food. Yes, the thing even pooped! This animated creation is where that popular phrase originated. Known as the "Duck test," it became the system we now call abductive reasoning (or deductive reasoning), the ability to draw conclusions from observation. You may be wondering what (if anything) does this have to do with food, much less the differences between GMOs and organic foods? Well, follow along, and you'll see.

While on a walkthrough of a Monsanto laboratory in St. Louis, Missouri, Vice President George H.W. Bush (then under President Reagan) verbalized that he would support deregulation of the genetically engineered foods industry. When the question of regulatory concerns came up, Bush replied, "Call me, I'm in the dereg. business—I can help!" The year was 1987. Two years later, Bush was the President of the United States and made good on his promise. He created the White House Council on Competitiveness on March 31, 1989, and delegated oversight of it to his Vice President, Dan Quale. Together, they double-handedly deregulated many industries, much to the detriment of the American people. Under these unconscionable practices, Monsanto, one of the largest agri-chemical/biotechnology companies, was able to monopolize the agricultural industry. Food and farming, as the world had known it, would never be the same. Most private and family farms were run out of business. From then up to now, the farmers who have managed to survive are being sued and tied up in all sorts of litigation by Monsanto. Monsanto always wins! To date, they have won judgments totaling close to 100 million dollars from these smaller farmers.

The deregulation of the agricultural industry under Bush and Quale didn't happen in a vacuum but was more than likely a byproduct of the seizure of family farms that began under the Reagan administration. But I digress. That's a whole story in and of itself. However, what happened was not only shocking but also was an ethical travesty. It was probably criminal.

Monsanto was literally allowed to monitor, self-police, and regulate itself! The Environmental Protection Agency (EPA), the Department of Agriculture (D Ag), and even the Food and Drug Administration (FDA) had no control or oversight of Monsanto's practices. The FDA only offered loose "guidance" and permitted "voluntary consultations" on safety matters. It was made evidently clear during the speech Quale delivered on May 26, 1992, that the special interest groups and the lobbyists for Monsanto had, in fact, gotten everything they wanted from the "deregulator-in-chief." This was the day that food, as we knew it, would never be the same again! From that moment on, consumers would very quickly be sold chemically and genetically engineered "foods," and farmers all across the country (and now, most of the world) would suffer under the litigious tactics, bullying, and worse from Monsanto.

The acronym GMO stands for genetically modified organisms.[1] In other words, living things whose genes and natural genetic composition have been manipulated to produce clones of the authentic food item that it looks like. Proprietary chemicals and biotechnological science are used to grow these products. Most of these items have either no seeds or have seeds that are sterile, meaning that they will not reproduce when planted. These seeds are called terminator seeds. Pesticides are built into them to automatically repel insects. Not only is this wholly unnatural to the way that food grows (natural pollination), but also the pesticides can be harmful to the human body. Some of the lawsuits levied against the farmers previously mentioned are to force farmers to use these GMO seeds, and therefore, the chemicals needed to grow them. These GMO products are known to cause diseases to organic crops when cross-contamination occurs.

With their arsenal of handsomely compensated lawyers, GMO producers also fight tooth-and-nail in our court systems against food labeling! Many entities and health-centric organizations that advocate for consumers' right-to-know have pushed for proper labeling of products. They believe and argue that people have a right to know what they are buying and feeding their families. The

---

[1] 'GMO-Free Non-GMO," Netherland Bulb Company. accessed October 4, 2020. https://www.netherlandbulb.com/index.cfm/fuseaction/home.showpage/pageID/199/index.htm.

GMO giants have spent tens of millions of dollars to fight them every step of the way!

Healthy eating is imperative for us to be strong. Being as optimally healthy as possible is critical as we attempt to do all we can to fight off COVID-19 and other viruses and diseases. This means that we need to consume real foods that provide our bodies with the vitamins, minerals, and nutritional benefits they provide. Although GMO products may look and may even taste like what it looks like, they often lack key nutritional elements. Is it any wonder that so many Americans have deficiencies in their bodies? Is it any wonder why so many Americans need to take all kinds of vitamins and supplements? It is not an overstatement to say that the time is now to be as vigilant as possible about your health. Consuming real (organic) foods in proper portions will have a tremendous effect on your health.

The cost of organic produce, dairy, and meat is slightly more expensive than GMO products. And yes, it is sometimes not as easily accessible. However, it is a small price to pay for the benefit of your health.

So, just because something looks like a duck, swims like a duck, and quacks like a duck, doesn't mean that it's a duck! The same is true for a watermelon. As we continue to go through this COVID-19 pandemic (and cold and flu season), being intentional about consuming real food—organic foods—is critical.

# CHAPTER 6: NATURAL HERBS AND SPICES AND THE AILMENTS THEY TREAT

C OVID-19 is the most daunting pandemic facing the world right now. But it is far from the only existential threat of which people need to be aware. There are many well-documented viruses, coronaviruses, diseases, and conditions that could become a crisis at any time. Yes, even another global epidemic or pandemic could occur simultaneously, as we are yet battling the pandemic of COVID-19. We've heard it said that education is our best defense. Although that is a true statement for most things in life, just knowing how to protect ourselves from COVID-19 and other viruses isn't going to be enough. This health crisis requires action. People are going to have to do something to guard and protect themselves and their loved ones. Hand washing, hand sanitizer, masks, and social distancing is good. They work, but they are external practices.

We must begin to build up our bodies and our immune systems to ward off these infections from within. Our bodies need to be an atmosphere that repels and is an unfavorable host to these viruses!

Statistics say that there are approximately twenty-seven million Americans without health insurance. That is almost ten percent of the population. This is a healthcare crisis within a healthcare crisis when you think about it. Hospital emergency rooms and ICUs (intensive care units) are at their breaking point with patients. They often operate without enough beds and equipment. Doctors and hospital staff have had to choose who they can treat and who they cannot. They have had to choose who they will try to save and who they must leave to die. For the least healthy who end up in the hospital, the odds aren't very good. It is safe to assume that those who haven't benefited from preventative care because of a lack of health insurance may be in that number.

There are myriad reasons that so many are uninsured. They include unemployment, under-employment, pre-existing health conditions that allow health insurers to refuse coverage, systemic and institutionalized racism that has had a generational, socioeconomic impact on people of color, and the like. Poor people and the 'working poor' of every ethnicity are greatly affected by the lack of health insurance and access to quality healthcare. Until our nation chooses to address these inequities substantively, this problem will always exist. This is not only unfortunate but is also unjust.

Until then, people need to educate themselves about and begin to practice practical and holistic measures to improve their health. The following is a condensed guide of natural and readily available elements to add to their personal arsenal against COVID-19 and other viruses. A key for the abbreviations is listed below the table.

| Anti-Viral Herb | Viruses/Conditions It Fights |
|---|---|
| Garlic | Influenza A & B, HPV, HSV-1, Rhinovirus, Viral Pneumonia, Rhinovirus, HIV |
| Clove | HSV-1 |
| Oregano (oil) | Norovirus, Rotavirus, MNV, HSV-1, RSV |
| Ginger | RSV, Avian flu, Norovirus |
| Rosemary | Influenza, HepA, HSV, HIV, HSV |
| Peppermint (leaves & oil) | RSV (and is also an anti-inflammatory) |
| Sage | HIV, HSV-1 |
| Thyme | HSV-1, HSV-2 |
| Basil (Holy) | HSV, HepB, Enterovirus, Avian Influenza |
| Fennel | HSV (and is also an anti-inflammatory) |
| Lemon Balm | HSV, HIV-1, Enterovirus |
| Ginseng | RSV, HSV, HepA, HepB, Norovirus |
| Dandelion | Influenza, HIV, HepB |
| Goldenseal | Influenza (H1N1) |
| Echinacea | Influenza, HSV |
| Licorice | SARS-CoV* (pneumonia), RSV, HSV, HIV |
| Sambucus (Elderberries) | Influenza, Rhinovirus (fights upper respiratory infections) |
| Astragalus | HSV, HepC, Avian Influenza |
| Turmeric | An anti-inflammatory and antioxidant that prevents heart disease, fights cancer, arthritis, and depression. It needs black pepper for absorption. |
| Cinnamon* (oil) | Antiviral Essential Oil |
| Bergamont* (oil) | Antiviral Essential Oil |
| Lavender* (oil) | Antiviral Essential Oil |
| Lemongrass* (oil) | Antiviral Essential Oil |
| Thyme* (oil) | Antiviral Essential Oil |

*Check for ingestion safety. Not all essential oils can be ingested!

Key:

- HepA/HepB/HepC - Hepatitis
- HSV1/HSV2 - Herpes Simplex Virus
- RSV - Respiratory Syncytial Virus (mostly affecting infants and children)
- HPV - Human Papillomavirus (leads to cervical and other cancers)
- HIV/HIV-1 - Human Immunodeficiency Virus (The virus that causes AIDS)
- MNV - Murine Norovirus
- SARS-CoV* - Severe Acute Respiratory Syndrome
- Influenza - The Flu (various strains)
- Rhinovirus - The Common Cold
- Norovirus - Often called 'Food Poisoning' or a 'Stomach Bug'
- MERS* - Middle Eastern Respiratory Syndrome
- SARS CoV2* - Corona Virus
- Avian Flu - (Bird Flu) H5N1
- Swine Flu - (Pig Flu) H1N1
- Rotavirus - Gastroenteritis (caused by fecal-oral contact)

*Indicates a Coronavirus

Vitamins and minerals, as well as other natural items, are vital for your body's health and strength. The following are a few that are very important to add to your self-care regimen to help your body fight or recover from viral invasions.

- Zinc helps the body fight off viruses and bacteria and is necessary to produce proteins and DNA.

40

• Vitamin D helps to build and fortify muscle tissue and cells. Every survivor of COVID-19 tells of the extreme muscle fatigue and pain they experience.

• Vitamin C helps the body fight the common cold virus.

• Chlorella is an incredibly nutrient-rich algae high in protein, vitamins, and minerals. It is a powerful antioxidant that rids the body of toxins and contains all of the essential amino acids.

• Chlorophyll supports the immune system, detoxifies the body, combats odor, and many believe it prevents some cancers.

This is a guide of the most common conditions and readily available herbs, vitamins, and minerals. This is not a fully comprehensive list of viruses, coronaviruses, and natural treatments.

*Christy Lopez*

# CHAPTER 7: REMEMBERING EBOLA

In March of 2014, the world became aware of a looming crisis that quickly became an epidemic in West Africa. This crisis was Ebola, a highly contagious and extremely deadly virus with a mortality rate of 90%. President Barack Obama and his team, led by former Ambassador to the United Nations turned National Security Advisor, Susan Rice, took action to prevent Ebola from becoming a pandemic in the United States. With a budget of only five point four billion dollars, medical teams and the US military were deployed to the affected areas in West Africa. The goal was to stem the global spread of the deadly Ebola virus by keeping it contained, fighting it on its own turf if you will. During this epidemic, there were 28,616 cases of Ebola globally, resulting in 11,310 deaths. There were five deaths in Europe and only two deaths in the US. The rest were all contained within six West African nations. Due to President Obama's leadership and an administration that were all on one accord, what could have become a devastating pandemic was stopped in its tracks!

There was a total of eleven cases of Ebola treated here in the US. One was a man named Thomas Duncan. He traveled to Dallas, TX, after visiting family in West Africa. He fell ill and was diagnosed and treated for Ebola at Dallas Presbyterian Hospital. Sadly, he lost his battle on October 8, 2014. Two nurses that treated Mr. Duncan, Amber Vincent, and Nina Pham, contracted the virus. Ms. Pham was airlifted to the National Institutes of Health (NIH) in Bethesda, MD, and Ms. Vincent was airlifted to Emory University Hospital in Atlanta, GA. They were both treated by teams of infectious disease doctors at their respective hospitals, and they both recovered.

Dr. Kent Brantley and Nancy Writebol both contracted the virus while working as missionaries in Liberia, while Dr. Ian Crozier was doing the same in Sierra Leone. They each became infected and were brought to Emory for treatment as well. They too recovered. The other Ebola patients were evacuees from other countries who were brought to Emory University Hospital for treatment. Emory was ground zero for treating this virus because of its physical and professional proximity to the Centers for Disease Control (CDC), headquartered in Atlanta, and because of its Serious Communicable Disease Unit (SCDU). Remarkably, there were only two deaths, though this virus has a 90% death rate. Protocols established because of the successful treatment of these critically ill patients have "evolved into internationally recognized standards for caring for patients with deadly infections," according to Emory University.[2]

President Obama and his National Security Council left the current administration a sixty-nine-page document titled, The Playbook for Early Response to High-Consequence Emerging Infectious Disease Threats and Biological Incidents. This "pandemic playbook" chronicled the successful plan of action

[2] "Five years later, Ebola patients return to Emory." Emory University. accessed October 4, 2020. https://news.emory.edu/features/2019/08/ebola-fifth-commemoration/index.html.

and implementation of procedures responsible for preventing Ebola from devastating us here in America or becoming a global crisis. Also left in place was a Pandemic Preparedness Office with a Pandemic Response Team established to respond to looming outbreaks around the world. This team was led by Ron Klaine, the "Ebola Czar."

Let's put a pin right here!

# CHAPTER 8: COVID-19: THE SYMPTOM

A s a nation, and globally, we are really living in strange days. The COVID-19 pandemic has illuminated many challenges and unmitigated failures in every societal system in America (Government, Media, Education, Economy, Religion, Family, Arts, and Entertainment). We can now clearly see just how interconnected one system is to another and the catastrophic results that resound when crucial decisions are being made without consideration for this interconnectedness.

Much can be said about the life-altering effects of the many failures that COVID-19 has exposed. Let's touch on a few.

Our economy is in shambles.

Between March and July of 2020, unemployment in America hovered just above 17%. By the numbers, over thirty million citizens were without jobs. This was the reported data, although the actual numbers would have reflected much higher had self-employed people, gig workers, and undocumented and migrant workers been included in a standard manner state to state.

The gravity of the pandemic brought our nation to a screeching halt. Our economy tanked in a free-fall, the likes of which haven't been seen since the great depression! With no income and no jobs to be found, thirty million of our fellow Americans were without the ability to pay their rent or mortgages. Car payments and insurance, utility, and other bills went unpaid as well. Health insurance lapsed, and lines snaked for blocks and miles on end as tens of millions of people were now dependent on food banks for just enough food to feed their families for a couple of days. Overnight, millions became destitute. Their ability to provide their families' most basic needs dried up along with their jobs. Whatever funds they had was all the funds they were going to have for months! As our government continues to devolve in its dysfunction, nearly forty million people are facing eviction and becoming homeless!

The inability to pay rent and mortgages is an obvious result of widespread unemployment. Although there was a federal and state moratorium on evictions in some cases, it isn't indefinite. When it expires, and it will expire at some point, families will face multiple months of back-rent. And many will still have no job or substantial income. Widespread homelessness is an existential threat that could become an epidemic within the pandemic.

Our education system is critically wounded.

To say our education system was "hard-hit" is an understatement, as daycares, schools at every level, and colleges and universities were shut down. Students from coast to coast and abroad were scrambling for flights home before airlines grounded nearly their entire fleet. Every school across the nation was thrust into the unchartered territory of having to educate students outside of school buildings. Creating and implementing distance learning has been a nightmarish undertaking, as the needs and socioeconomic backgrounds of students are so varied. The risk of regression for students is great—even greater for children with special needs, as parents and caregivers struggle to teach them.

Of an estimated fifty-six million students in the US in grades K-12, 14% do not have internet access at home, and 17% of students do not have a computer in the home. It is reported that 4% of school-age students live in areas where internet service isn't even available! It goes without saying that lower-income and children living in poverty, as well as poor rural areas, are affected the most by the lack of access to technology. This problem is exponentially worse in homes with siblings, regardless of the age group, because the need for computers is multiplied. These are grim statistics for nine and a half million children. Let that sink in.

Our government is guilty of malpractice.

The worsening of the pandemic, the increase in loss of life, the crippling of our economy, and the education system are all direct results of having failed leadership in the White House. Equally culpable, however, are the members of Congress and the Senate who have enabled it all along the way. They turned a blind eye to the destruction and degradation of our constitution and allowed "#45's" dereliction of duty to continue. They've turned blind eyes and waved white flags of surrender, allowing "#45" to continue to run roughshod over our country. They have given him a green light at every intersection of corruption and treason.

The country watches as congressmen and senators use verbal jiu-jitsu to deny and plead the fifth to ignore the dismantling of our country at every turn. The inch given has now become a country mile taken, and the consequences are incalculable to every dimension of humanity and are laying the cornerstone to an authoritarian government—a dictatorship.

Yet, government leaders aren't the only ones responsible for the crisis we're experiencing.

The church has become a blasphemous adulterer!

Religious leaders—certainly not all but—most acutely evangelical "Christians," which I would punctuate with a lowercase c, also have a hand in this nation's failings. They have not only sat idly by but have propped up and excused such poor leadership. They've exclaimed that "#45" and his policies are righteous, and even go so far as to say that he is a decent "Christian" man (again, I would punctuate with a lowercase c). They, too, have turned blind eyes, but in this case, it is to every teaching of God through Jesus, with the exception being pro-life. Contorting themselves and the word of God in the Bible to support a wicked leader! The evangelical church has gone from detesting and admonishing those lacking family values, to those lacking decent character, and at least an appearance of a wholesome moral barometer, to now fully supporting and defending "#45's" lack thereof! The evangelical church has decided that the fruit of the Spirit, according to Galatians 5:22-23, doesn't apply to "#45," but rather the works of the flesh in Galatians 5:19-21 are perfectly acceptable attributes for a so-called God-fearing leader. The truth of the matter is that the evangelical church sect is simply revealing who they genuinely are. They are using a twisted interpretation of scripture related to honoring authority to be open and blatantly culpable in supporting hateful and destructive policies, most of which are steeped in racism. They are justifying their racism and hate for the foreigner under the cloak of honoring governmental authority, and are willingly grieving God, Jesus, and Holy Spirit by cheerleading "45's" morally and ethically bankrupt antics. How incredibly sad. How utterly consequential.

Sadly, other church leaders have chosen to stay silent or have failed to speak up and oppose the misrepresentation of the church and Christ's teachings by the sect. The Jesus the evangelical church teaches about would never be happy with the same evangelicals' thoughts, words, deeds, and twisting of his teachings, laws, commandments, ordinances, and statutes. The behavior and lack of decency they support, and their excuse doesn't square at all with real Christian values.

The horrific toll that COVID-19 has taken on our economic and educational system is a direct result of a careless, callous, and inept leadership in both the executive and legislative branches of government. There are no checks and balances.

No one can deny that the 45th president has been a total and complete failure across the board, but especially in the mismanagement of this pandemic! He has failed miserably at handling this crisis from the very beginning, insisting that it will simply "go away." His initial lie to the American people was that the first few reported cases in Washington State were in people that were "recovering nicely." On February 10, 2020, he falsely claimed that it will go away in April with the heat. On February 26, 2020, he stated that there are fifteen people with it, and in a few days, " it'll be close to zero." The very next day, he said that it (the virus) would "just disappear...that it'll just be a "miracle." On March 6, 2020, and again on March 10, 2020, he admonished us to "be calm" that the virus was just going to go away. On March 17, 2020, (six days after the WHO did so) "#45" finally declared COVID-19 a pandemic. Although the entire world watched and heard him downplay its severity for months, he then stood in the White House briefing room and said, "I've always known—this is a—this is a real —this is a pandemic—I've felt it was a pandemic long before it was called a pandemic—all you had to do is look at other countries...I've always viewed it as very serious."

Had he always known that it was a pandemic, why did he sit back and literally do nothing? Why constantly undermine scientific data and the expertise of Dr. Anthony Fauci, our nation's leading infectious disease doctor?

Again on March 31, 2020, he stated that the virus was "going to go away at the end of the month...maybe even before that." Many more times (too many to mention), he continued with his constant refrain of blatant lies and wishful thinking that COVID-19 would just go away, even referring to coronavirus many times as a "democratic hoax."

On May 24, 2020, it was reported that the coronavirus has claimed 100,000 lives.

Let's take the pin out from where we stopped in the previous chapter entitled Remembering Ebola.

*Remembering Ebola Continued*

To recap, in March of 2014, the world became aware of a looming crisis that quickly became an epidemic in West Africa. This crisis was Ebola, a highly contagious and extremely deadly virus with a mortality rate of 90%. President Barack Obama and his team, led by former Ambassador to the United Nations turned National Security Advisor, Susan Rice, took action to prevent Ebola from becoming a pandemic in the United States. With a budget of only five point four billion dollars, medical teams and the US military were deployed to the affected areas in West Africa. The goal was to stem the global spread of the deadly Ebola virus by keeping it contained, fighting it on its own turf if you will. During this epidemic, there were 28,616 cases of Ebola globally, resulting in 11,310 deaths. There were five deaths in Europe and only two deaths in the US. The rest were all contained within six West African nations. Due to President Obama's leadership and an administration that were all on one accord, what could have become a devastating pandemic was stopped in its tracks!

President Obama and his National Security Council left the current administration a sixty-nine-page document titled, The Playbook for Early Response to High-Consequence Emerging Infectious Disease Threats and Biological Incidents. This "pandemic playbook" chronicled the successful plan of action and implementation of procedures to prevent exactly what we are living through right now, the COVID-19 pandemic. Also left in place was a Pandemic Preparedness Office, with a Pandemic Response Team that President Obama established to respond to looming outbreaks around the world. This team was led by Ron Klaine, the "Ebola Czar." Ebola became neither an American nor a global crisis.

The Pandemic Response Team conducted tabletop exercises with the incoming administration after the 2016 election. The team kept America safe from the threat of infectious diseases until they were each fired or otherwise dismantled by "#45's" National Security Advisor in May of 2018. The rationale for getting rid of our first line of defense against threats of devastating viruses and diseases was never made clear. Neither was there any attempt to reassemble them once it was evident that COVID-19 was quickly becoming the pandemic it is today.

These points are being highlighted for those who shamefully choose to believe the lies and false accusations against President Obama that have come from the current occupant of the White House. President Obama has no responsibility for the 100,000 plus lives lost due to COVID-19. The revisionist history and "alternative facts" are known to most people as good old-fashioned big fat lies! It has threatened our democracy and our national security. Facts matter. These are the facts. You're welcome!

Contrast that with these hard facts:

Over 100,000 people in the US are dead. Trillions of dollars were spent in economic stimulus money, corporate bailouts, and corrupt lending. Now, weigh the fact that none of this money has done anything substantive to stop the spread of COVID-19. Remember the daily pleas of doctors, nurses, and frontline workers in hospitals and skilled care facilities all across this nation who were literally begging for PPE. (Remember them having to reuse the N-95 masks they did have)! Remember when "#45" stood in the White House and said of the government, "We're not a shipping clerk," in response to states' need of federal stockpiled materials or acquisition of materials? Remember the time he boldly admitted that he was refusing to give much needed federal aid to states whose governors aren't nice to him or who don't shower him with appreciation? And he admonished his VP not to communicate with governors who don't treat him right. All the while, people were dying.

Remember when masks, state closures, and re-openings were politicized and cost even more lives. Think back on his refusal to invoke the Defense Production Act (DPA) in a timely manner for companies to start making ventilators and much-needed materials such as PPE or virus testing kits.

The list of failures and unconscionable negligence of the current administration is well documented. Those who continue to support and defend the failed policies of the executive branch and its leader know well that "#45" is unfit for the office in every way! For some empty reason, they continue to do so even to their own detriment. Why? It has cost so many people their lives. It has literally ruined this country and destabilized the world.

As the name of this chapter states, COVID-19 is the manifested symptom of the actual sickness of this country. The disease of apathy. The infection of racism. The virus of unchallenged corruption. The cancer of injustice. All these left untreated for so long has created a smelly, septic open wound. Our beloved nation and our democracy will soon die if we do not deal with these atrocities once and for all. This pandemic is a wake-up call to those choosing to operate in malpractice and with a disregard for basic truth and decency. We can no longer afford to stand by and allow blind partisanship rooted in greed and hateful ideology to govern this land. It is literally killing us!

It is for these reasons that *Pandemic Solutions: How to Fight COVID-19 and Other Coronaviruses* was written. As we are living in a day and age where every system norm is broken, and that we need to be equipped with the knowledge and tools to help ourselves. Getting healthy and staying healthy by building a strong immune system is imperative. It's impossible to overstate the importance of incorporating natural foods and herbal remedies into your diet and lifestyle. Do it as if your life depends on it. It just might.

Be well.

## COMING SOON

# *The Pandemic Solutions Recipe and Cookbook*

*The Pandemic Solutions Recipe and Cookbook* features healthy, tasty, and simple meals and drinks, and incorporates nature's most potent ingredients.

It is a beautiful bounty of well-balanced meals that are easy to prepare, good for you, and as delicious as they are aesthetically pleasing. Let's eat to live and enjoy it!

And be sure to follow me on Facebook for more information at https://www.facebook.com/Pandemic-Solutions-112203530631984/.

*Christy Lopez*

# ABOUT THE AUTHOR

Ms. Christy Lopez is a highly regarded and super-talented hairstylist, makeup artist, and salon owner in the Washington, DC area.

Raised by her loving maternal grandparent, on a farm in the small town of Gambrills, MD, Christy's life reflects two of her primary early childhood influences, beauty and nature. Her grandmother, Mrs. Mamie Turner, would style hair at home, creating enviable hairstyles for local women and family members. This sparked an incurable interest in the world of beauty. Her grandfather, Mr. John Turner, would garden, harvesting every fruit and vegetable in its due season, as well as canning, preserving, hunting, and raising pigs and chickens. This is where her love of nature began.

Christy has worked at every level in the beauty industry, from her first job of being a shampoo-girl to salon ownership. She has maintained a steady and racially diverse clientele throughout the years and is a master in every aspect of hairstyling.
There's nothing she can't do. Clients come from near and far to have their hair styled; a few have even boarded planes or driven for hours to sit in her chair!

Her expertise and professionalism have led to many notable editorial experiences in the media, styling hair and doing makeup for many outlets and entities. The highlight of her career was working in the hair and makeup department for CNN in the political bureau in Washington, DC. There, she was trusted to style world-renowned and globally recognized news anchors, journalists, politicians, and celebrities. This was an awesome experience for Christy, who once dreamed of going to college to become a broadcast journalist, a dream long deferred.

After many years as a dedicated mom raising her son into adulthood, working diligently in the local church, singing and leading worship, and being a dutiful friend and encourager to others, Christy is now in a season of rediscovery of her God-given gifts, talents, and dreams. She has found excitement and purpose in pursuing them unapologetically, come what may!

She enjoys spending quality time with her son through their traditions of playing jeopardy, super-competitive games of scrabble, watching movies, and binge-watching Law & Order SVU. Her hobbies include cooking, trying new foods, and swimming.

For more information, visit https://www.facebook.com/Pandemic-Solutions-112203530631984/.

.

*Christy Lopez*